DOWN SYNDROME

THINGS YOU SHOULD KNOW

(QUESTIONS AND ANSWERS)

By Rumi Michael Leigh

Introduction

I would like to thank and congratulate you for purchasing this book, " *Down syndrome, things you should know (questions and answers)*" series.

This book will help you understand, revise and have a good general knowledge and keywords of Down syndrome.

Thanks again for purchasing this book, I hope you enjoy it!

Table of Contents

Section 1

1) What is a syndrome?

- A syndrome is a combination of signs and symptoms related to one another.

2) Is Down syndrome a genetic disorder?

- Yes, Down syndrome is a genetic disorder.

3) Is Down syndrome a common genetic disorder?

- Yes, Down syndrome is a common genetic disorder.

4) Can Down syndrome be inherited?

- Yes, Down syndrome can be inherited.

5) Is Down syndrome always inherited?

- No, Down syndrome is not always inherited.

6) What is the prevention of Down syndrome?

- Down syndrome cannot be prevented.

7) Down syndrome is also called?

-   Down syndrome is also called Trisomy 21.

Section 2

1) What is a chromosome?
- A chromosome is a long DNA molecule that contains the genetic material.

2) What is a gene?
- A gene is a DNA fragment.

3) What are the sex chromosomes?
- The sex chromosomes are the X and Y chromosomes.

4) What are the male chromosomes?
- The male chromosomes are the X and Y chromosomes.

5) What are the female chromosomes?
- The female chromosomes are the XX chromosomes.

6) How many chromosomes ae there in the cell of a human body?

- There are 46 chromosomes in the cell of the human body.

7) How many pair of chromosomes does the human body have?

- The human body has 23 pairs of chromosomes.

8) What is the cause of Down syndrome?

- Down syndrome is caused during abnormal cell division that results into an extra chromosome 21.

9) Is the extra chromosome 21 always a full chromosome?

- No, the extra chromosome 21 is not always a full chromosome. It could be a partial chromosome.

10) How many copies of chromosome 21 is there in the cells of a person with Down syndrome?

- In a person with Down syndrome, there are 3 copies of chromosome 21 in the cells.

Section 3

1) What is aneuploidy?
- Aneuploidy is an abnormal chromosome number.

2) What is hypoploidy?
- Hypoploidy is a few chromosome numbers less than the normal chromosome numbers.

3) What is hyperploidy?
- Hyperploidy is a few chromosome numbers greater that the normal chromosome numbers.

4) What is meiosis?
- Meiosis is cell division.

5) What is a cell?
- A cell is the basic unit of an organism.

6) What are gametes?
- Gametes are the reproductive cells in an organism.

7) What is the male gamete?

-   The male gamete is sperm.

8) What is the female gamete?

-   The female gamete is the ovum.

9) A person with Down syndrome has how many chromosomes?

-   A person with Down syndrome has 47 chromosomes.

Section 4

1) What is mutation?

- Mutation is a change in DNA sequence.

2) Are autosomes sex chromosomes?

- No, autosomes are not sex chromosomes.

3) What are the sex chromosomes?

- The sex chromosomes are the X and Y chromosomes.

4) How many autosomes are there?

- There are 22 pairs of autosomes.

5) How many heterosomes are there?

- There is 1 pair of heterosome.

6) Heterosomes are also called?

- Heterosomes are also called sex chromosomes.

Section 5

1) What is monosomy?
- Monosomy is one copy of a chromosome in a diploid cell instead of two copies.

2) What is nullisomy?
- Nullisomy are missing copies of the same chromosomes.

3) What is polysomy?
- Polysomy are extra copies of chromosomes.

4) What is nondisjunction?
- Nondisjunction is the failure of correct chromosomes separation.

5) How many trisomy is there in nondisjunction in meiosis one?
- There is two trisomy in nondisjunction in meiosis one.

6) How many trisomy is there in nondisjunction in meiosis two?

- There is one trisomy in nondisjunction in meiosis two.

7) What is a haploid cell?

- A haploid cell is a cell that contains one set of chromosomes.

8) What is a diploid cell?

- A diploid cell is a cell that contains two sets of chromosomes.

9) What is the male sex cell?

- The male sex cell is the sperm.

10) What is the female sex cell?

- The female sex cell is the egg.

Section 6

1) What is the normal number of copies of chromosome 21 in the cells of an individual?

- The normal number of copies of chromosome 21 in the cells of an individual is two.

2) How many chromosomes are usually donated by a father?

- 23 chromosomes are usually donated by a father.

3) How many chromosomes are usually donated by a mother?

- 23 chromosomes are usually donated by a mother.

4) Is there only one type of Down syndrome?

- No, there is not only one type of Down syndrome.

5) What is Mosaic Down syndrome?

- Mosaic Down syndrome is a form of Down syndrome where there are the extra copies of chromosome 21 present in some cells.

6) What is translocation Down syndrome?

- Translocation Down syndrome is a form of Down syndrome where the chromosome 21 is attached to another chromosome.

7) Can translocation in Down syndrome be inherited from parents?

- Yes, translocation in Down syndrome can be inherited from parents.

8) Is the severity of Down syndrome the same in people?

- No, the severity of Down syndrome is not the same in people. It may vary from one person to another.

9) What are the signs and symptoms of Down syndrome?

- The signs and symptoms of Down syndrome include short stature, a small head, protruding tongue, small hands, small feet, epicanthal fold, special facial features, oblique eye fissure, cognitive problems, small ears, short neck, simian crease, brachycephaly, nystagmus, clinodactyly, Brushfield's spots, excess skin in neck, intellectual disabilities, congenital heart disease, etc.

10) What are the complications of Down syndrome?

- The complications of Down syndrome include immune disorders, leukemia, obesity, heart problems, gastrointestinal problems, problem with the spinal cord, dementia, sleep apnea, hypothyroidism, infections, epilepsy, duodenal atresia, otitis media, etc.

Section 7

1) What is an epicanthal fold?

- Epicanthal fold is a skin fold of the upper eyelid that covers the inner corner of the eye.

2) What is microcephaly?

- Microcephaly is an abnormal small baby head size.

3) What is simian crease?

- Simian crease is the line across the palm of the hand in an individual.

4) Normally, how many transverse simian palmar creases are there?

- Normally, there are two transverse palmar creases.

5) How many transverse simian palmar creases are there in a person with Down syndrome?

- In a person with Down syndrome there is normally one transverse palmar crease.

6) What is brachycephaly?

- Brachycephaly is an abnormally shaped anteroposterior skull of an infant.

7) What is nystagmus?

- Nystagmus is a condition that causes involuntary rapid movement of the eye.

8) What is clinodactyly?

- Clinodactyly is an abnormal curved finger.

9) What are Brushfield's spots.

- Brushfield's spots are colorful spots around the iris of the eye.

10) What is endocardial cushion defect?

- Endocardial cushion defect is a congenital heart condition. This is a malformation or absence of the walls that separates the upper and lower chambers of the heart.

Section 8

1) What is leukemia?

- Leukemia is cancer of the blood and or the bone marrow.

2) What is polycythemia?

- Polycythemia is a condition that causes an increase in the red blood cells.

3) Polycythemia is also called?

- Polycythemia is also called polyglobulia.

4) What is sleep apnea?

- Sleep apnea is a disorder that causes a person to stop breathing and restart breathing during sleep.

5) What is hypothyroidism?

- Hypothyroidism is an insufficiency of the production of thyroid hormones.

6) What is hypotonia?

- Hypotonia is a low muscle tone.

7) What is otitis media?

- Otitis media is the inflammation of the middle ear.

8) What is epilepsy?

- Epilepsy is a disorder due to an electrical disturbance in the brain.

9) What is hypoplasia?

- Hypoplasia is an underdevelopment of an organ or tissue.

10) What is duodenal atresia?

- Duodenal atresia is an obstruction of the duodenum due to congenital malformation.

11) What is Hirschsprung disease?

- Hirschsprung disease is a congenital condition that affects the colon. It prevents stool from passing.

12) What is a popular congenital heart disease in a person with Down syndrome?

- A popular heart disease in a person with Down syndrome is atrioventricular septal defect.

Section 9

1) What are the risk factors for Down syndrome?

- The risk factors for Down syndrome include a woman having children with advancing age, and being a carrier.

2) What is the biggest risk factor for Down syndrome?

- The biggest risk factor for Down syndrome is maternal age.

3) Can a woman less than 35 years old give birth to a child with Down syndrome?

- Yes, a woman less than 35 years old can give birth to a child with Down syndrome but the risk is far less than a woman older than 35 years.

4) Are most men with Down syndrome infertile?

- Yes, most men with Down syndrome are infertile.

5) Are most women with Down syndrome infertile?

- No, most women with Down syndrome are not infertile.

6) What is the cure for Down syndrome?

- There is no cure for Down syndrome.

7) Are there treatment options for Down syndrome?

- Yes, there are treatment options for Down syndrome.

8) What are the treatment options for Down syndrome?

- The treatment options for Down syndrome include speech therapy, physical therapy, occupational therapy, etc.

Section 10

1) Can Down syndrome be diagnosed?

- Yes, Down syndrome can be diagnosed.

2) Can Down syndrome be diagnosed during pregnancy?

- Yes, Down syndrome can be diagnosed during pregnancy.

3) What is the diagnosis of Down syndrome?

- The diagnosis of Down syndrome includes screening tests and diagnostic tests.

4) What is chorionic villus sampling?

- Chorionic villus sampling is a medical test done during pregnancy where a sample of chorionic villus is taken from the placenta in order to check for abnormalities.

5) What are the levels of estriol in a mother with a fetus with Down syndrome?

- In a mother with a fetus with Down syndrome, estriol levels are lower than in a mother with a fetus without Down syndrome.

6) What is estriol?

- Estriol is an estrogen hormone.

7) What produces estriol?

- Estriol is produced by the placenta.

8) What is amniocentesis?

- Amniocentesis is a medical test that involves taking a sample of the amniotic fluid in a pregnant woman.

9) What is percutaneous umbilical blood sampling?

- Percutaneous umbilical blood sampling is a medical diagnostic test that examines blood from the umbilical cord.

10) Percutaneous umbilical blood sampling is also called?

-   Percutaneous umbilical blood sampling is also called cordocentesis.

11) What is Karyotype?

-   Karyotype is the analysis of chromosomes.

12) What is an ultrasound?

-   An ultrasound is a medical test that uses sound waves to create images of the body.

13) Is pre-natal screening test an accurate diagnostic of Down syndrome?

-   No, pre-natal screening is not an accurate diagnostic of Down syndrome but it helps to evaluate the risks of Down syndrome.

14) Is the diagnostic test more accurate for the diagnostic of Down syndrome compared to the pre-natal screening?

-   Yes, the diagnostic test is more accurate for the diagnostic of Down syndrome.

Conclusion

Thank you again for purchasing this book. I hope it has helped you in your journey to understanding Down syndrome.

Please, if you enjoyed this book, I would like you to rate and comment. It'd be appreciated.

Thank you.